8 Secrets About Teeth
EVERYONE
Needs to Know

to Save Money, Time & Grief

TED GRELLNER DDS

ISBN-13: 978-1533697677
ISBN-10: 1533697671

Dr. Ted Grellner
Theodore J. Grellner DDS, PA
Oral & Maxillofacial Surgery
15310 Amberly Dr
Suite 195
Tampa, Florida 33647

PH: **813-972-3478**
Email: tg@grellnerdds.com
website: grellnerdds.com

Media Inquiries:
Email: ted@drtedgrellner.com
website: www.drtedgrellner.com

Printed in the United States of America

DEDICATION

This book is dedicated to all
who wish to keep their teeth for a lifetime.

DISCLAIMER

This book is intended as an educational document and is not to be considered as dispensing specific medical or dental advice to you.

The author and the publisher shall have neither liability nor responsibility to any person or entity with respect to any loss, damage, or injury caused or alleged to be caused directly or indirectly by the information contained in this book.

The information presented herein is in no way intended as a substitute for medical/dental counseling or medical/dental attention.

Table of Contents

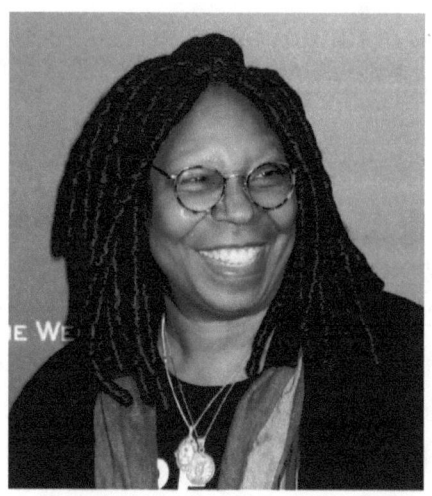

Introduction

Whoopi Goldberg almost lost her front teeth due to gum disease that caused severe bone loss.

John Glascock, bass guitarist & vocalist for the band **Jethro Tull**, died at age 28 because of a congenital heart defect made worse by a tooth abscess.

Both situations resulted from neglecting <u>routine</u> dental problems! People don't realize that REALLY bad things can happen if you don't take care of your teeth.

This book is for anyone who has teeth in their mouth, and wants to keep them for as long as possible.

"8 Secrets About Teeth EVERYONE Needs to Know", contains information YOU don't know – but need to know - about the dental issues you can encounter over your lifetime, as well as other issues you may experience with the passing of time.

In this book are "<u>secrets</u>" dental professionals learn as a result of dealing with people who constantly struggle with their teeth.

No one wants to smile with holes in their teeth or spaces where teeth have been lost prematurely to cavities or gum disease.

Worse yet is trying to smile with slipping dentures because you lost all your teeth at a very young age.

To many, it seems impossibly difficult to avoid dental problems.

The quicker you start using the secrets in this book, the slower that dental problems will develop, the less pain you may have to endure from those problems, the less risk you may face dealing with your teeth down the road, and the longer you may be able to keep your teeth.

Keeping teeth for a lifetime is certainly not out of the question.

This book was intentionally kept short and non-technical so that you can absorb the information in it quickly.

Putting these tips to work for you can potentially **save you** a lot of **money, time, and grief**.

The information in this book will bring some "Ah-ha" moments helping you to better understand dental issues, enabling you to make smarter decisions about your teeth at every stage of your life.

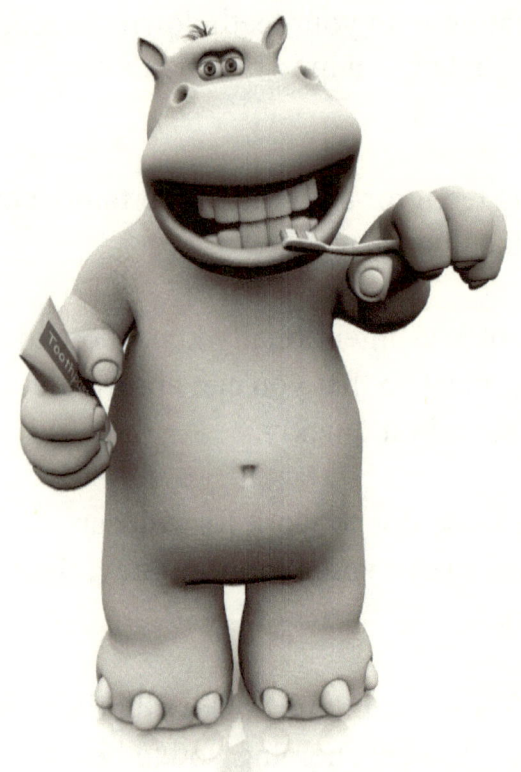

The 1ˢᵗ Secret

The 1ˢᵗ Secret is that <u>how often</u> you brush your teeth is less important than <u>how many minutes</u> you have processed <u>sugar</u> in your mouth.

Have you ever heard someone complain that even though they brush their teeth 3 or 4 times a day, they keep getting cavities with absolutely no idea as to why?

Or there's the person who does more than "just" brush their teeth. They have the skill, desire and time to really take meticulous care of their teeth and gums, making them much cleaner than the first person's. And yet even they will still get occasional cavities despite their excellent hygiene.

Then you see a third person who scrubs his teeth back and forth with a brush, as if he were shining his shoes, ignoring all the nooks and crannies between the teeth. And, of course, *he* is the one who rarely gets a cavity.

What's going on here? We'll get to the answer shortly.

While some blame their cavities on having inherited soft teeth or bad bacteria from their parents, you can't change what you inherit, can you? So let's forget these factors you can't control.

Let's approach this from an angle that you **can** actually do something about.

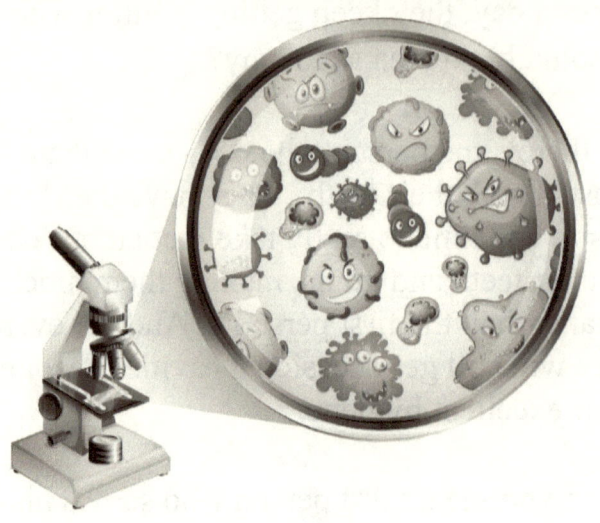

<u>Bacteria</u> …

… that cause cavities are microscopic - so small that we can't see them. The ability to remove something that numbers in the millions (or billions) on your teeth, that you can't see or get to, is understandably an impossible task.

The first two people feel that they work hard to get the cavity-causing bacteria off their teeth; one brushing more often than needed but not as well as he could, the other being much more thorough, and yet they <u>both</u> get cavities.

Why?

They are both <u>missing the very same places</u> every time they brush so when they eat sugar, providing food for the bacteria they leave behind, cavities form right in those missed places.

How can you possibly eliminate an enemy you can't see or get to?

Hmmm…

Then the third guy, the one with the poorest brushing technique, gets many fewer cavities

---- because <u>he hardly eats any sweets</u>.

Voila! (as the magician would shout!) Could this be your answer?

If you can't possibly remove <u>all</u> the cavity-causing bacteria, why not attack the problem differently with something you <u>can</u> do - by <u>reducing what you feed the bacteria</u>? Starve the little bast_rds! (Their only goal in life is to harm your teeth)

<u>Are you saying that I have to give up all sweets?</u>
No, absolutely not. Like dieting, giving up

ALL sweets would never work because realistically you wouldn't be able to stick to it.

But, what you CAN do is **limit the _TIME_ that <u>sugar</u> is in your mouth** – feeding the bacteria less well - thus slowing the rate that cavities form.

<u>How will this work?</u>
Think of the bacteria sticking to your teeth as little processors that turn sugar into acid.

The longer they have sugar available to process into acid, the longer that acid will be in contact with the tooth.

Since you've probably seen what happens when acid gets on things, you can picture your tooth slowly breaking down where the acid touches it.

The tooth surface exposed to the acid will first turn chalky white, then crumble away to form a cavity (hole in the tooth).

This roughened/hollow surface on the tooth will now trap even more bacteria because your brush and floss won't be able to reach them in the hole, so the destruction accelerates.

Getting back to those the first two people who got cavities despite their frequent or thorough brushing - they probably paid no attention to how much time they had something sugary in their mouths.

While presweetened cereals, sodas, candies and desserts are obvious sources of sugar, there are so many others that are less so, like the sugar added to the coffee or tea they drink or processed foods with added sugar they eat, or the peppermints they might unconsciously suck on while working.

The average American consumes WAY MORE sugar than they realize - would you believe the equivalent of a 5 lb. bag of sugar every 10 days?! (150-170 lbs. per year per USDA (U.S. Dept. of Agriculture))

But the cavity problem isn't as dependent on how much sugar you consume, but rather how much **TIME** sugar stays in your mouth to be converted into tooth-destroying acid.

You could have a HUGE piece of birthday cake once a day and have fewer cavities than one who consumes sugared drinks, mints or even worse: a few caramels – over a longer period of time.

The Secret
Limit your sweets to non-sticky forms that you can eat/drink relatively quickly. Better yet, rinse with water right afterwards to dilute or remove any sweetness that remains.

The worst offender is a sweet that sticks to your teeth for long time, like a caramel, before it finally dissolves away.

With sugar, the key is the TIME it is in your mouth. Think of starting a stopwatch when you start consuming a sweet and stopping it when the sweetness in your mouth is gone after rinsing.

Then, imagine restarting that stopwatch every time you put something sugary sweet into your mouth.

The less accumulated time on your virtual stopwatch, the fewer cavities you will get.

While you still need to <u>clean your teeth as thoroughly as you can at least once a day</u> to remove as many bacteria from your teeth and gums as possible, you now have way to slow your cavity rate that is actually do-able.

BONUS – <u>**FAILING CROWNS**</u>

Ever wonder why your crowns ("caps") seem to fail in what seems like only a few short years after they were put in?

They fail most often because of cavities that form where the crown margin meets the tooth.

Since you know that cavities result from acid-forming bacteria that remain in areas where you can't clean, why are crown margins so vulnerable?

The answer is based on the different "worlds" in which we and those pesky microscopic bacteria live.

While the dentist and lab technician who made your crown were working on a macroscopic level (what is visible to the naked eye), the bacteria in your mouth live in a much, much smaller world, the microscopic level (where you need a microscope to see them).

Though the margin where the crown joins your tooth may feel smooth and closed to these dental personnel, it's going to appear to bacteria as a HUGE gap where they can easily accumulate.

Since you can't get to the bacteria effectively with your brush or floss, they will feast on all the sugar you put into your mouth until the ledge they live on starts to enlarge into a room (the cavity).

Since most crowns are made of materials like metal that x-rays can't penetrate, a new cavity won't be seen until it gets large enough to destroy the part of the tooth below the crown margin. As a result, these cavities often can't be found until they are quite large.

Once the deep cavity approaches the center of the tooth, pain begins – the topic of our next Secret!

How do you prevent these cavities? Again, if you can't see or get to your invisible enemy to remove them, be smart and deny the bacteria what they thrive on: SUGAR!

Hopefully then, you will be able to extend the life expectancy of your crowns, bridges, and fillings. That would be quite a money saver!

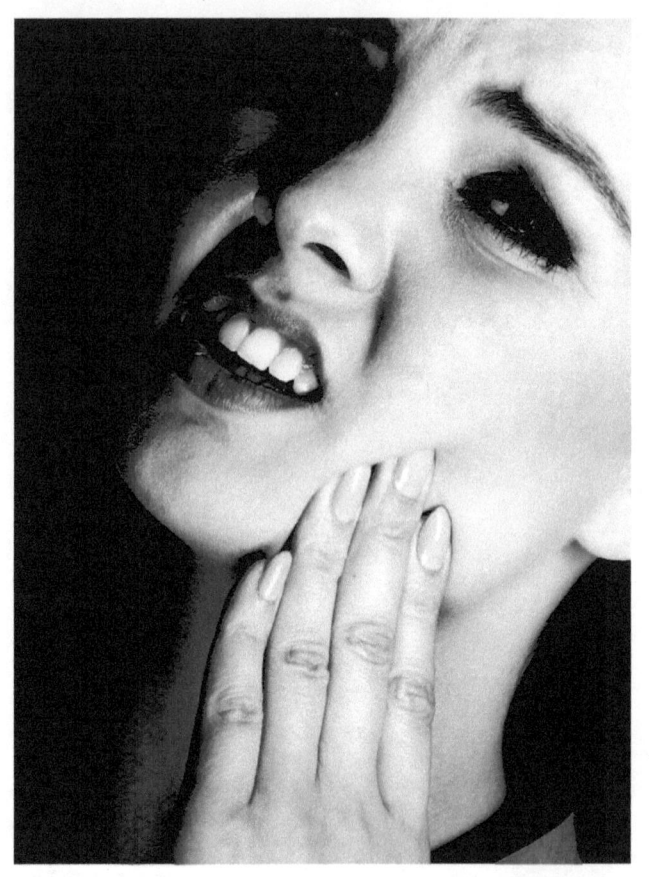

The 2nd Secret

The **2nd Secret** is that **once a cavity begins to cause <u>pain</u>, it will probably take more than just a filling to fix it.**

Toothache pain generally means the bacteria in the cavity have started to infect the inside of your tooth – now requiring either a root canal or extraction to eliminate the source of the infection.

To ignore this pain is to risk the infection getting worse, sometimes much worse.

Yes, it might temporarily go away for a while without treatment, but don't be fooled into thinking that it went away for good. It WILL return, sometimes with a vengeance, especially when your immune system becomes compromised by another form of infection like a flu or cold.

The reason untreated tooth infections come back, unlike a sore throat, is that the hollow insides of the tooth & its roots hide the infecting bacteria from your immune system.

Since the dead, infected tooth no longer has an active blood supply to bring in your immune cells or antibiotics to kill the bacteria, your body has no way to fight the infection inside.

The tooth needs to be cleaned out and roots sealed at their end (a root canal), or the tooth removed entirely, to do away with this reservoir of bacteria that can flare up at any time.

WORST CASE SCENARIO
Infections from teeth can sometimes turn into a life-threatening process that can overwhelm your body's defenses so severely that you could need emergency surgery and care in an ICU (intensive care unit).

When a tooth infection gets out of hand, spreading to the face, throat and/or neck, it can cause a brain abscess or so much swelling and pus that the airway (the tube that carries air down to your lungs) could be narrowed, or even closed by the pressure on it.

Treatment of big infections like these can involve drainage of the infection from inside and outside the face and neck to relieve the pressure on the airway and other vital structures, and IV antibiotics to try to kill the bacteria causing the infection, which can sometimes take a week or more.

While big infections like these are uncommon, ANY infection in your mouth, be it a tooth infection, gum infection around a wisdom tooth, etc. has the potential to get out of hand, especially if ignored long enough.

One clue to how severe your infection may become is how RAPIDLY it is getting worse.

Once you have developed severe difficulty opening your mouth, or especially swallowing or breathing, you have waited too long to get your infection under control with only oral antibiotics.

These progressively worsening symptoms mean that you need to be seen by an oral surgeon quickly; don't wait to get in with your family dentist. If you don't have an oral surgeon you can call, you'd best get to the emergency room of a local hospital that has one on call.

Of course, if your symptoms have progressed to emergency status, call 911 for help rather than risk driving yourself to the hospital.

Returning to the tooth that has just started to hurt …
Needless to say, ignoring tooth or gum pain is risky. While gum pain could be minor enough

to resolve itself without treatment, tooth pain is a different story.

Though the infection causing the toothache might get better for a while without treatment, it will inevitably return, often worse than before. You should **never** ignore a toothache.

A word about pain relief
While **aspirin** is a good pain reliever and was the only non-prescription product available until meds like ibuprofen, acetaminophen, etc. came along, it causes a lot more bleeding with surgery because it permanently disables the platelets in the blood, preventing them from sticking to form a clot. That's why physicians initially put their patients on only a ¼ tablet daily to thin the blood.

If you are taking aspirin as a pain reliever only, stop it 5-7 days before any possible surgery – this is how long it takes for your body to make new functioning platelets to replace the ones you knocked out with the aspirin.

If a physician has you on aspirin daily, call him first before discontinuing it.

More important than pain relief for a toothache, though, is <u>getting an antibiotic</u> that can <u>temporarily</u> control the cause of your pain - the infection - until you can get it treated.

The bottom line on toothaches
If you want to minimize costs, time lost and grief maintaining your dental health, you need to catch dental problems when they are small, less damaging and much cheaper to fix.

Once a tooth starts to ache, your problem is now a far bigger one. The cost to treat your ailing tooth (root canal + crown, OR extraction + bone graft + dental implant + crown) is going to be significantly greater than a filling done earlier when the cavity was much smaller.

Since cavities don't cause pain until they become larger, and form in areas you can't always find on your own, <u>regular visits to your family dentist,</u> to catch those cavities when they are small, <u>are a must</u>.

Regardless of whether you have dental insurance or not, the cost for regular exams, cleanings and small fillings is far less than fixing the damage of neglect later.

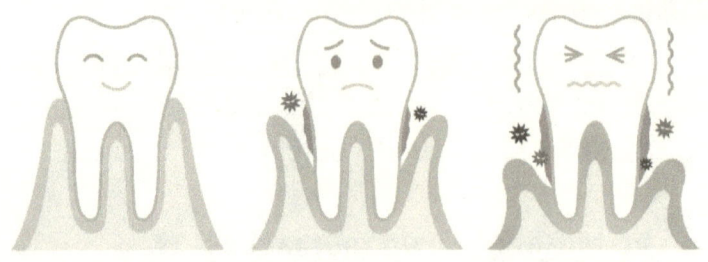

The 3rd Secret

The **3rd Secret** is that <u>gum pain</u> *can* signal a **gum infection** which can melt away the bone holding a tooth.

Surprisingly, this could happen <u>within days</u> (like when a popcorn kernel gets deeply stuck in your gum!).

While this is an **acute** form of gum infection, most people may not notice the slower, subtler, **chronic** form of gum disease (referred to as periodontal or gum disease) until years later when their teeth start to loosen, like Whoopi's situation with her front teeth.

Regular visits to your general dentist are important to monitor and treat early signs of gum disease before too much bone is lost.

<u>Bone is the precious hard tissue</u> that is needed to firmly support your teeth in your jaw for chewing.

Avoiding the loss of bone is also important if you would like to replace a tooth (that can't be fixed) with an implant. This is especially important in the front of the mouth where there is less bone to begin with.

Bone will melt away quickly when exposed to bacteria in the form of an acute infection, more slowly when the infection is less aggressive, but it will also melt away in a situation where infection is not even present! (Secret #5)

According to the CDC (Centers for Disease Control), **smoking** weakens the immune system's ability to fight off infection and gum disease. Smokers have <u>twice the risk</u> for gum disease than non-smokers.

The Academy of General Dentistry reports that a one-pack-a-day smoking habit can cost you the loss of at least two teeth every 10 years!

Information is now coming out in Europe that low blood levels of **vitamin D** can accelerate bone loss as well.

Read up on Vitamin D. You will find that it is an incredibly important vitamin to maintain at healthy levels, with careful sun exposure or by supplementing (preferably with vitamin D3).

Read up on Vitamin K2. Recent information suggests that K2 works with Vitamin D to improve absorption of calcium, slows arterial calcification and directs calcium to the bones.

Ask your physician about proper dosing of these vitamins and to help monitor your blood levels of vitamin D so you're getting enough, but not too much.

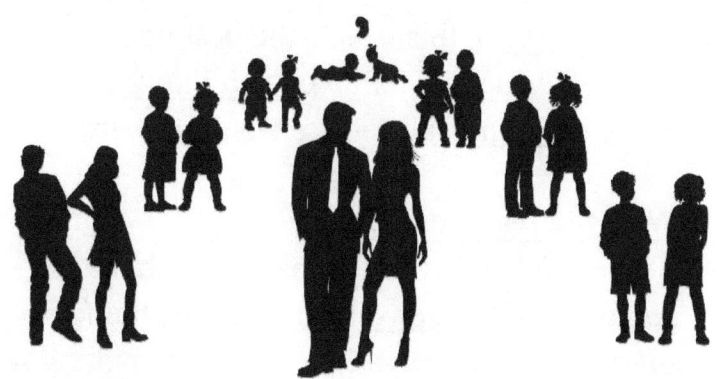

The 4th Secret

The **4th Secret** is that **tooth removal from healthy bone is easiest in the mid-teens**.

As much as parents still think of their teens as kids - since it seems like just yesterday when they were – they're rapidly maturing into young adults on their way to adulthood.

While we seem to only pay attention to the physical changes we see on the outside, little do we think about what's going on <u>inside</u> their bodies as well.

So, why would you take a tooth out of healthy bone?

While teeth are often removed when younger to make room for an orthodontist to straighten

crowded teeth, this is also the best opportunity
Nature gives us to remove teeth likely to
cause problems later – like **wisdom teeth**.

Why the teen years?
Because a teen's soft, immature jawbone is
going to harden considerably in just the few
short years between ages of 15 - 20, making it
much harder to remove teeth after 20.

An analogy would be comparing what it
might be like to rock a fence post out of dirt
that has been softened by a week of rain (teen
bone) vs. rock-hard, sun-dried dirt (adult
bone). The difference can be that dramatic.

Any experienced oral surgeon will agree that
this factor alone makes wisdom tooth removal
much easier, thus less traumatic, in the teens
than later in the 20's.

BONUS

While there are many other reasons why the
teen years are the best time to remove wisdom
teeth, there is one more very important
advantage that teens have (that adults have
lost): shorter, **immature roots**.

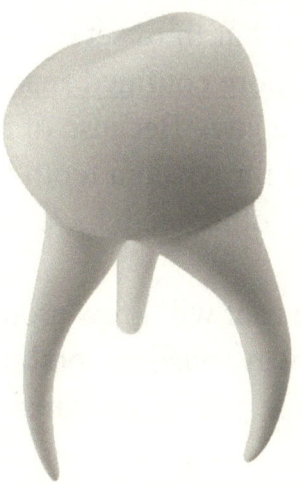

As the roots of a multi-rooted tooth grow (like the molar above), several different things can happen to make that molar harder to remove later. The roots can grow:

- Longer
- Not parallel to each other
- Curved rather than straight
- Narrower and more fragile in their lower half
- Bulbous (locking them into the bone like a round onion)

The closer the roots get to completing their growth (maturity), the harder any of these factors will make the removal of the tooth.

The area in the back of the jaw, where the wisdom teeth (our third set of molars) grow, is a <u>smaller, more confined space</u> than further forward in the jaw. Because of this, it is not at all unusual for wisdom tooth roots to curve, even if all the other teeth have straight roots.

Just as a tree root will grow around a hard object in its way, wisdom tooth roots will also grow along the path of least resistance.

It also seems that the roots will keep growing until reaching the length pre-determined by your genes, whether there is room for that full length or not.

A wisdom tooth root can even double back upon itself or turn to the side when there isn't room for it to keep growing straight.

The advantage to removing <u>immature</u> wisdom teeth is that there's much less resistance to removal when the roots are short and straight.

Don't allow the difficulty to increase by letting the roots grow to their full length.

So, <u>the most ideal time to remove wisdom teeth</u> is when:

1. they sit in softer, immature bone
2. their roots have not matured

These 2 factors alone will provide a much better experience for your teen than later as an adult.

This ideal opportunity to evaluate and remove the wisdom teeth starts in the mid-teens. It is a once-in-a-lifetime event in the lifecycle of the wisdom teeth that will silently come and go without you ever being aware of the advantages that it briefly offered.

What age is best?
It varies a lot between kids. Wisdom teeth can be completely formed by age 15 or only just starting to form their roots by 19 - it can vary that much.

The most important thing is to catch them **before** they (the wisdom teeth) finish growing.

It's best to start looking early, then plan accordingly based on the progress of their growth.

Unless your child's teeth came into the mouth later than other children, we suggest parents bring their teens in for a wisdom tooth evaluation around age 15 or so.

If the panoramic x-ray we take reveals that their wisdom tooth roots have not yet started to form, it may actually be more difficult to remove them at that point.

We'll reassess perhaps in a year or two, to determine when it would be easiest and best to remove the wisdom teeth.

The Key is TIMING.

Much more information on wisdom teeth is available on my website:

http://www.grellnerdds.com/oral-surgery/wisdom-tooth-removal

Two more quick thoughts:

The harder the surgery is for the surgeon, the more difficult the recovery will usually be for the patient.

…and….

How often have you seen a teen <u>heal *slower*</u> than an adult from the same surgery?

Enough said?

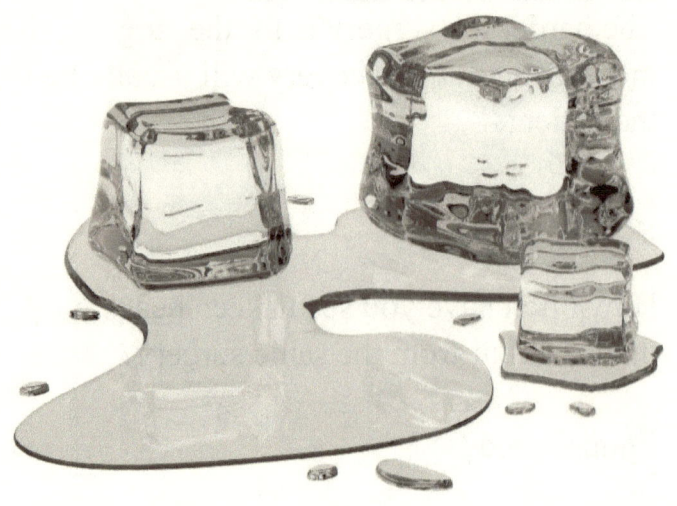

The 5th Secret

The **5th Secret** is that **the bone of a <u>healing</u> adult tooth socket is,** in fact, **<u>already</u> starting to disappear!**

What?!!

While the tooth socket - where the roots of your recently extracted adult tooth used to be - will be filling in with new bone as it heals, the <u>outer</u> <u>surface</u> of the socket bone will already be starting to slowly melt away like an ice cube!

This process occurs with <u>every</u> tooth you lose - a very important process to be aware of when you decide to have a decayed but restorable tooth removed rather than repaired.

When a <u>single adult tooth</u> is lost …
… the bone of the healed socket will begin to narrow and shorten in height - until years later when it feels to your finger as if the bone has completely melted away.

If this isn't bad enough, in the back of the upper jaw where the sinus lies next to the roots of the upper molars, the sinus itself will begin to creep down into the missing tooth socket, melting away bone from above!

The bone then actually disappears from both directions because there are no roots to maintain its width and height and keep the sinus in place. Isn't this crazy?

<u>So what do you do?</u>
The only way to slow this natural process of bone loss is to replace the missing tooth root(s) with a dental implant about 2-6 months later, adding bone to replace what may have already melted away.

Usually an implant is placed after some bone healing has already taken place to hold the implant securely (an implant won't bond to the bone properly if it is loose).

Sometimes it may be possible to place an implant the same day your tooth is extracted, but many argue that there is added risk to doing so.

The dental implant serves two purposes:
1. Holds a crown for chewing
2. Transfers bite forces, generated by chewing, back into the bone to replicate what the previous tooth root(s) did. This stimulation helps to preserve the bone where the implant is, slowing further bone loss.

When all the adult teeth are removed …
… and replaced with dentures, this bone loss process occurs where every tooth has been lost.

Infection is not the cause of this spontaneous bone loss (though it can certainly cause additional loss of bone), nor does the pressure of the denture on the jaw ridge seem to cause it - it happens even when dentures are never worn.

Many oral surgeons have <u>a demonstration plaque</u> in their office that has 4 plastic jaw models mounted to it.

These adult jaws dramatically demonstrate the process of **"the disappearing jaw"**, the progressive loss of jaw bone after the adult teeth are lost:

- a healthy jaw with all its teeth
- a jaw just after all teeth have been removed
- a jaw showing bone loss after only 10 years
- a jaw with bone loss so severe that it has shriveled to almost the **size of a finger** in a frighteningly short **20-25 years**!

A person who has reached this end-stage of bone loss is truly a dental cripple because they can no longer wear a denture.

People who still try are usually struggling to do so with lots of strong denture adhesive because there's no bone ridge left to keep the denture from sliding around. They either have to "gum" their food, or "blenderize" it beforehand.

What causes that "sunken" facial appearance in some older adults?

If you've ever wondered why the faces of people who have worn <u>dentures</u> for many years seem to have shrunk, this natural, progressive bone loss is the reason.

The jaws lose height and width, causing the lower face to collapse and recede inwards.

Rushing to dentures to avoid taking care of your teeth has long term consequences most people either don't know or think about.

Again, bone is the <u>precious</u> substance necessary to hold teeth, dental implants, and support dentures.

Bone is <u>not permanent</u>, and when not cared for it goes away with devastating consequences years later.

Chewing food is vital to our health, and a visibly healthy facial structure will ultimately depend on keeping our teeth and jaw bones.

To summarize, bone loss starts slowly in areas where bacteria cannot be reached for cleaning, but accelerates to much more rapid loss with acute infections of the gums or teeth.

And, as you've just learned, loss of bone continues even after you lose your teeth.

Good dental care is a lifelong investment that can become very expensive when small problems that have been ignored, turn into much bigger ones.

What is my Formula for Dental Success?

- Pick one time a day to clean your teeth <u>as thoroughly as you can.</u>

  In areas where you cannot remove bacteria trapped by teeth that are crowded or impacted, seek help in fixing these problems before bone loss or cavities appear.

- Reduce the **time** that **sugary sweets** are in your mouth

- Get regular dental exams (and cleanings) to <u>catch problems when they are small</u> and less expensive to fix; bigger problems bring much bigger expenses.

  Doing these things will help considerably to preserve your teeth and supporting bone much longer.

  The alternative? Having to soak your "teeth" in a glass at night while you sleep.

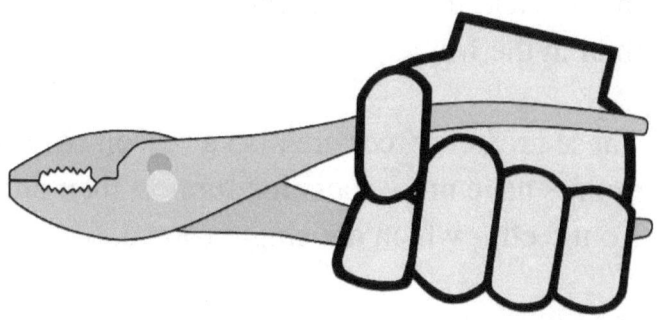

The 6th Secret

The **6th Secret** is that **the habit of clenching and grinding your teeth is not the <u>harmless</u> habit** you once thought it was.

Your jaw shares an important property with these pliers.

<u>But first, answer this question:</u>
"If you needed to grasp a bolt with the greatest force, would you grab it with the front or back of the pliers?"

You would do so with the <u>back</u> of the pliers closest to the hinge because this is where you can generate the most force.

Similarly, our jaws generate much more force in the back, the molar area closest to joint, than in the front.

These greater forces are also a reason why our molars have more roots for support than our front teeth - which are single rooted.

What you don't know
While you know that teeth will wear down when excessive grinding, what you don't know is that too often the back teeth can actually <u>break</u> under the heavy pressure of clenching.

Once split, infection will follow. The broken tooth will have to be removed because it can't be saved.

<u>Prevent this</u> by having your general dentist custom-make you a <u>heavy plastic night-guard</u> to protect your teeth from these destructive biting forces.

If you clench your teeth …
… **during the day** when you are stressed or in the gym lifting weights, you have your best chance to consciously stop it. For times when

you can't stop it, wear your nightguard to protect your teeth.

At night it is impossible to stop something you are unaware of doing, so the nightguard is especially important to wear then.

An added bonus of wearing a nightguard is reducing sideways pressures on any dental implants you may have, as you clench and grind.

Research shows that only the top 3-4 mm of bone supporting your implant receives the bulk of the chewing & grinding forces exerted on it.

If you grind/clench excessively, this bone at the top of your implant will start melting away circumferentially (all the way around it). If allowed to continue, you risk losing the implant prematurely.

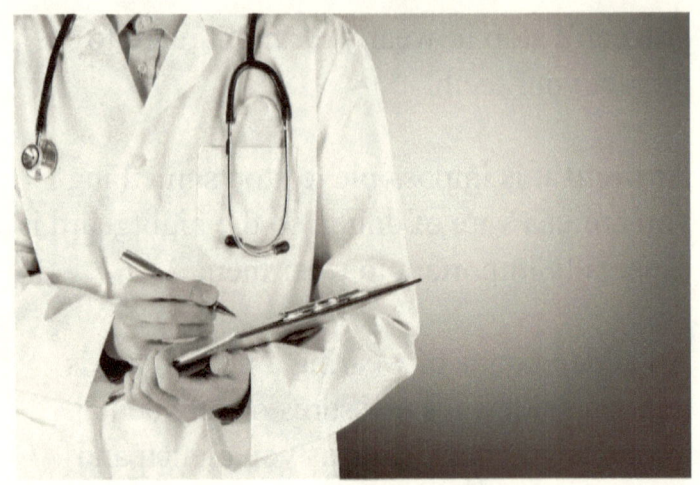

The 7th Secret

The **7th Secret** is that **medical issues can affect <u>needed</u> oral surgery treatment**.

<u>HIGH BLOOD PRESSURE</u>

High blood pressure (hypertension) <u>that is _not_ controlled</u> can possibly cause a stroke when undergoing a potentially uncomfortable or stressful procedure like a tooth extraction.

Although your tooth may be hurting, it is far safer to wait for your physician to control your hypertension with medication first.

Unfortunately, this could delay needed dental treatment <u>for weeks</u>. Attempting to reduce your pain with antibiotics is a temporary option.

HEART ATTACK

Heart muscle damaged by a recent **heart attack** (myocardial infarction) could take 6 months to heal sufficiently. Your cardiologist will decide when its safe for you to proceed with dental treatment.

Ignoring your medical AND dental health can put you in a situation where an important medical issue can delay treatment of the less important dental problem.

OSTEOPOROSIS

As a result of taking certain medications for **osteoporosis** (soft/weak bones) over several years, routine tooth extractions or other surgery on the jawbone may not heal properly without first taking a lengthy holiday from that medication - for as long as <u>6 to 12 months</u>!

Why? It takes more than <u>11 years</u> for only **half** of this medication, that has been incorporated into your bone, to break down and leave your system naturally.

Waiting 6 to 12 months for the drug level to correct enough to allow the bone to heal is a relatively short time in comparison.

These medications (known as bisphosphonates) are toxic to the bone cells called osteoclasts. These cells function like vultures to clean up damaged or dead bone to make room for new.

Since jawbone is unavoidably damaged by surgery as minor as a tooth extraction, it may not heal properly without sufficient functioning osteoclasts.

PREGNANCY
And finally, a very important concern for women is **pregnancy.** Pregnancy can affect the timing of dental treatment, limit the types of antibiotics and pain medication that can be prescribed, as well as the choices of anesthesia available to you, due to concern for your baby.

Pregnancy complicates dental treatment more than one would realize so make sure you're healthy dentally as well as medically <u>before</u> **risking** pregnancy.

Dealing with dental problems <u>after</u> discovering you're pregnant ~~can~~ <u>will</u> make for a much more difficult dental experience.

***

An example of what you might consider to be a "routine" dental problem complicated by pregnancy:

A 30-year-old woman in her 2nd trimester of pregnancy suddenly gets a painful wisdom tooth infection – the gum partially covering her impacted wisdom tooth is now badly infected.

Even though this is the 2nd or 3rd time she's had this problem ("they always went away before"), she never eliminated the problem by having her wisdom tooth removed, due to her fear.

1st Problem: Treat with antibiotics only?

Since this is a <u>recurring infection</u> - simply treating it with antibiotics will not be enough now.

The partially exposed wisdom tooth needs to be removed because bacteria is trapped where she cannot clean, risking the return of infection once off the antibiotic.

2nd Problem: Limited anesthesia choices

Removal of an impacted wisdom tooth from a fearful patient is much less stressful on her (and her baby) with a well-controlled deep sedation or general anesthetic. Obstetricians (OB's) typically prefer surgery performed awake using local anesthesia only.

If you were the pregnant patient in this example, could you do a difficult wisdom tooth extraction awake using only local anesthesia?

3rd Problem: Limited antibiotic choices

Soft tissue infections, like this gum infection around the wisdom tooth, need to be successfully treated <u>before</u> opening the gum to remove the tooth.

Operating on infected gum tissue risks active infection spreading into surrounding areas like the throat or neck if the prescribed antibiotic fails to treat it quickly enough (or at all).

This happens because lifting the gum away from the impacted tooth releases the boundaries that limit the spread of your infection. These tight boundaries buy time for your antibiotic to work.

Violate this principle by insisting that your tooth be removed - before confirming that the antibiotic has successfully treated your infection - risks you ending up in the hospital for stronger IV antibiotics and possibly surgery to drain pus from the infected areas. Not a pretty picture and certainly not a risk worth taking. (Note: the decision on how to proceed with your infection must be made by the surgeon managing your care because situations can vary).

The reason for emphasizing the importance of completely eliminating the gum infection around the wisdom tooth before removal is this: obstetricians initially limit you to narrow spectrum antibiotics like penicillin. Penicillin is not as effective against dental infections as it once was, especially against a long-standing or repeat infection.

OB's are reluctant to allow additional, or stronger antibiotics without being consulted first. This can increase your risk of infection worsening, delaying treatment.

4th Problem: Limited pain meds

OB's also prohibit a pregnant woman from taking an NSAID (non-steroidal anti-inflammatory drug like ibuprofen, naproxen sodium, etc.) for pain. Unfortunately, these meds are far more effective for oral surgery pain than the acetaminophen or narcotic you will be limited to.

You have to be a tough woman to handle this situation with all the limitations placed on it by the pregnancy and your doctor (no fault of the OB's – they're only trying to protect you and your baby as best they can).

As you can see, a "simple" wisdom tooth problem can become far more difficult once you realize all that is involved in treating it.

If you know you're a **dental "chicken"**, be smart and take care of all potential dental problems before chancing pregnancy, when you can do it much more comfortably and safely.

Your options become much more limited once that "+" sign appears on your urine test for pregnancy.

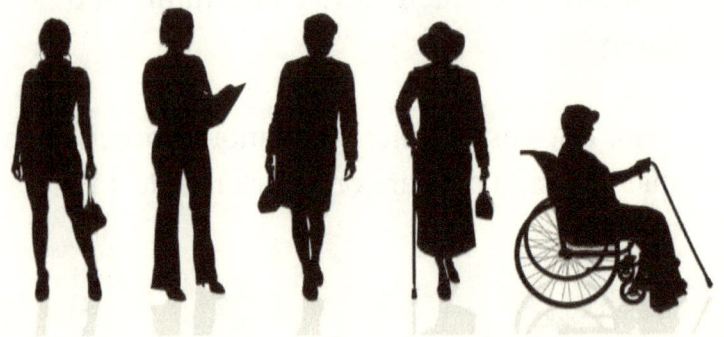

The 8th Secret

The **8th Secret** is a reminder that **dental problems don't retire when you retire.**

It anything, dental problems may worsen as your manual dexterity starts to decrease.

This may seem very obvious, yet people will simply disregard their dental health when they're older until dental issues worsen to the point they <u>can't</u> be ignored any longer.

While this can happen at all ages – it's human nature - you've gotten a hint in the last chapter how medical issues can interfere with getting needed dental treatment <u>when YOU want to get it</u>.

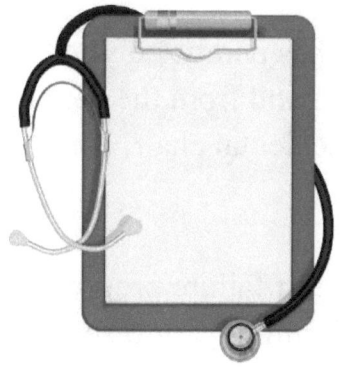

Medically more complicated and risky

What makes the situation <u>more difficult</u> when you postpone treatment <u>in your later years</u> is that you may have waited until medically it is <u>much more complicated and risky</u> to treat you than just a few years earlier.

As you get older your health may start to decline, often dependent upon how well you had taken care of yourself earlier.

Not to be negative, but there are so many potential issues that can interfere with getting dental treatment and even medical treatment:

- a <u>heart arrhythmia</u> now requiring blood thinners that must be managed carefully when it comes to dental surgery

- a <u>stroke</u> that has paralyzed you to the point that getting to and from the dental office, in and out of the dental chair, is now so much more difficult

- <u>congestive heart failure</u> progressively worsening, limiting your reserve or stamina. Your ability to tolerate stress, or to receive sedation for your procedure, is now diminished

- a <u>cancer</u> requiring chemotherapy that severely limits your ability to fight infection. A routine dental extraction may have to be postponed until your immune system recovers.

- <u>deteriorating mental awareness</u> (Alzheimer's Disease, for example) that can interfere with your acceptance and tolerance of dental treatment

- <u>lung disease</u> (like COPD – chronic obstructive pulmonary disease – that makes it more difficult for you to breathe effectively) now prevents you from being deeply sedated for an oral surgical procedure

- a newly discovered <u>throat or mouth cancer</u> requiring radiation treatment that must be delayed until the decayed / infected teeth are removed and the jaw healed adequately

And these are just a few of the issues you could encounter.

Ignoring both your dental and medical health could put you into a position where you could literally be **risking your life** to receive even <u>routine</u> dental treatment.

<u>EXAMPLE</u>
You've put off a long-standing dental problem that has now escalated into what you consider to be a dental emergency (a tooth, that has been bothering you on and off for months, now hurts <u>constantly</u> and <u>severely</u>).

You have also been ignoring intermittent chest pain that has now progressed to unstable angina (chest pain that comes on <u>*without* any cause to initiate it</u>). This could potentially be life-threatening if you fail to tell your dentist about it and try to receive dental treatment without treating the heart problem first.

Just as teens should prepare for adulthood by eliminating potential dental problems early, it's even more critical that seniors not ignore small problems that may turn into bigger ones in their later years, be it dental or medical.

Like the Boy Scout motto advises: <u>Be Prepared</u> – so you can better enjoy your Golden Years!

Conclusion

Congratulations on getting to this point, the conclusion of this short book.

My son, the business man, tried to warn me against writing this book saying that no one would ever read a book about teeth.

By getting here, you have not only proven him wrong, but your reward for doing so is having gained valuable information that can benefit you for the rest of your life IF you put the 8 Secrets to use.

Since memory thrives on repetition, on the next page is a quick review of the 8 Secrets.

Review the Secrets

The **1**st **Secret** is that <u>how often</u> **you brush your teeth is less important than** <u>how many minutes</u> **you have processed** <u>sugar</u> **in your mouth**.

The **2**nd **Secret** is that **once a cavity begins to cause** <u>pain</u>**, it will probably take more than just a filling to fix it.**

The **3**rd **Secret** is that <u>gum pain</u> *can* signal a **gum infection** which can melt away the bone holding a tooth.

The **4**th **Secret** is that **tooth removal from** <u>healthy</u> **bone is** <u>easiest</u> **in the mid-teens**.

The **5**th **Secret** is that **the bone of a** <u>healing</u> **adult tooth socket is,** in fact, <u>already</u> **starting to disappear!**

The **6**th **Secret** is that **the habit of clenching and grinding your teeth is not the** <u>harmless</u> **habit** you once thought it was.

The **7**th **Secret** is that **medical issues can affect** <u>needed</u> **oral surgery treatment**.

The **8th Secret** is a reminder that **dental problems don't retire when you retire.**

The Review After the Review

If you found this book to be particularly valuable, others will as well.

If you would be so kind as to take just a few minutes to go to Amazon to recommend this book, I would be immensely honored and grateful.

Thank you.
TG

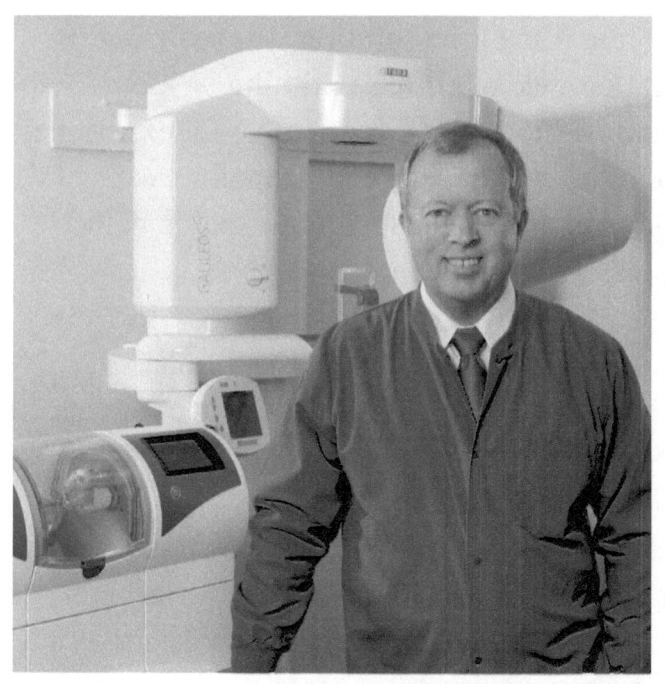

The Author

Tampa Oral Surgeon Dr. Ted Grellner, as a college student, endured a bad experience with a wisdom tooth.

Little did Dr. Ted know then that he would be pursuing a career in dentistry, to discover multiple ways to improve the oral surgery experience so his patients could avoid what he suffered through.

While part of the solution was realizing the importance of correctly timing wisdom tooth removal to create a more pleasant experience, another was developing a quick recovery IV general anesthesia technique that is both pleasant and safe.

For lost or missing teeth, Dr. Ted has incorporated the digital accuracy of advanced computer technology into the placement of dental implants.

Dr. Grellner has 30 years of experience in oral and maxillofacial surgery (OMFS) and is a Courtesy Clinical Assistant Professor in the Dept. of OMFS at Univ. of Florida College of Dentistry in Gainesville, Florida.

He has appeared on ABC, FOX and NBC stations to share his dental expertise.

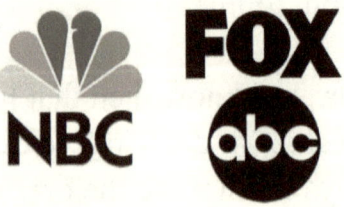